# A SEX EDUCATION GUIDE FOR PARENTS

## An ultimate Guide to Conversations about Sex with Your Child

### FELICIA AKINS

# CONTENTS



How to Talk to Your Child About Sex

## INTRODUCTION

As parents, we want our children to grow up healthy, happy, and safe. We talk to them about good manners, the importance of education, and the dangers of drugs and alcohol. But when it comes to sex, many parents feel uncomfortable or unsure about how to approach the topic with their children.

It's understandable to feel apprehensive about having "the talk." Maybe you're afraid of saying the wrong thing or giving too much information. Perhaps you're worried that your child will be embarrassed or uncomfortable. Or maybe you're uncomfortable with the topic of sex yourself.

However, avoiding conversations about sex can have serious consequences. Studies have shown that children who receive comprehensive sex education from their parents are more likely to make informed and responsible decisions about sexual behavior as they grow older. Children who do not receive such education are more likely to engage in risky sexual behavior, have unintended pregnancies, and contract sexually transmitted infections.

Moreover, talking openly and honestly about sex can help build trust and strengthen your relationship with your child. When you create a safe space for your child to ask questions and express concerns, you're building a foundation of trust and communication that will serve you both well throughout their lives.

It's important to understand that sex education isn't a one-time conversation. It's an ongoing dialogue that evolves over time as your child grows and develops. By starting the conversation early and continuing it throughout your child's life, you're helping to create a healthy and positive attitude towards sex and relationships.

In this book, we'll provide you with the tools and strategies you need to talk to your child about sex in a way that is age-appropriate, respectful, and informative. We'll address common fears and misconceptions about having "the talk," and we'll show you how to create an open and supportive environment for these important conversations. By the end of this book, you'll feel confident and empowered to have ongoing conversations with your child about sex, relationships, and their bodies.

Talking to your child about sex can be a daunting task for many parents. There are a variety of common fears and misconceptions that can make it feel like an overwhelming challenge. In this chapter, we'll address some of the most common fears and misconceptions and provide guidance on how to overcome them.

Fear #1: "I'll Give Too Much Information"

Many parents worry that they'll provide too much information and overwhelm their child. However, it's important to remember that children are curious and want to know about their bodies and how they work. It's better to provide accurate information rather than leaving your child to fill in the gaps with misinformation or harmful stereotypes.

Fear #2: "I'll Say the Wrong Thing"

It's natural to worry about saying the wrong thing or using the wrong language when talking to your child about sex. However, it's important to remember that honesty and openness are key. If you're unsure about something, it's okay to admit it and look up accurate information together.

Fear #3: "I'll Embarrass My Child"

Many parents worry that talking about sex will make their child uncomfortable or embarrassed. However, it's important to remember that creating a safe and supportive environment for these conversations can help to alleviate these feelings. Start with open-ended questions and let your child guide the conversation.

Fear #4: "My Child is Too Young"

Many parents worry that their child is too young to talk about sex. However, it's important to remember that sex education is an ongoing process that starts early. Children are curious and observant, and it's better to provide accurate information at an early age rather than waiting until they hear inaccurate information from their peers or the media.

Benefits of Having Open and Honest Communication with Your Child

Talking openly and honestly about sex can have numerous benefits for your child's physical and emotional health. When you provide accurate information and create a safe space for conversation, you're helping to promote healthy attitudes towards sex and relationships. Some of the benefits of having open and honest communication with your child about sex include:

- Increased knowledge and understanding about their bodies and how they work

- Increased confidence and self-esteem

- Better decision-making skills when it comes to sexual behavior

- Reduced risk of unintended pregnancies and sexually transmitted infections

- Stronger relationships based on trust and communication

In the next chapter, we'll explore the basics of sex education and provide guidance on how to approach age-appropriate conversations about sex and relationships.

# UNDERSTANDING SEX EDUCATION

Sex education is an important part of your child's development. It helps them to understand their bodies, develop healthy attitudes towards sex and relationships, and make informed decisions about their sexual health. In this chapter, we'll explore the basics of sex education and provide guidance on how to approach age-appropriate conversations.

## The Basics of Sex Education

Sex education encompasses a wide range of topics, including:

- Anatomy and physiology: Understanding the male and female reproductive systems and how they function.

- Gender and sexual identity: Understanding the differences between biological sex, gender identity, and sexual orientation.

- Healthy relationships: Understanding the characteristics of healthy relationships, including communication, respect, and trust.

- Consent: Understanding the importance of giving and receiving enthusiastic consent in sexual encounters.

- Safe sex: Understanding how to protect oneself from unintended pregnancy and sexually transmitted infections.

## The Importance of Age-Appropriate Conversations

It's important to remember that sex education is a process that evolves over time. Conversations about sex and relationships should be age-appropriate and tailored to your child's level of understanding. For example, a conversation with a five-year-old about anatomy and physiology might focus on basic body parts and functions, while a conversation with a teenager might include a more in-depth discussion of sexual health and safe sex practices.

## How to Approach Difficult Topics such as Consent and Safe Sex

Approaching difficult topics such as consent and safe sex can be challenging, but it's important to provide accurate and age-appropriate information. Here are some tips for approaching these topics:

- Consent: Start by talking about respect and boundaries in relationships. Explain that it's important to ask for permission before touching someone and that it's okay to say no to unwanted touch. Use examples that are relevant to your child's life, such as asking permission before borrowing a toy from a friend.

- Safe sex: Start by explaining the importance of protecting oneself from unintended pregnancy and sexually transmitted infections. Use age-appropriate language and provide clear and accurate information about how to use condoms and other forms of contraception.

Remember, open and honest communication is key when it comes to sex education. By creating a safe and supportive environment for these conversations, you're helping to promote healthy attitudes towards sex and relationships and empowering your child to make informed decisions about their sexual health.

# PREPARING YOURSELF FOR THE CONVERSATION

Talking to your child about sex can be a challenging and emotional experience, but it's important to remember that it's also an opportunity to provide valuable information and support. In this chapter, we'll explore how to prepare yourself for the conversation by dealing with your own discomfort and anxieties, identifying your values and beliefs about sex, and setting goals and expectations for the conversation.

## Dealing with Your Own Discomfort and Anxieties

It's normal to feel uncomfortable or anxious about talking to your child about sex. However, it's important to address these feelings before the conversation. Here are some tips for dealing with your own discomfort and anxieties:

- Educate yourself: Read books, watch videos, and talk to experts to help educate yourself about the topics you'll be discussing with your child.

- Practice: Practice what you want to say and how you want to say it. This can help you feel more comfortable and confident during the conversation.

- Address your own biases: Reflect on your own values and beliefs about sex and relationships. Identify any biases or stereotypes you may hold and work to overcome them.

Identifying Your Values and Beliefs about Sex

Before you have the conversation with your child, it's important to identify your values and beliefs about sex. These beliefs can influence how you approach the conversation and what information you provide. Some questions to consider include:

- What are my values and beliefs about sex and relationships?

- How do I feel about premarital sex?

- What are my expectations for my child's behavior?

- How do I want to talk about gender and sexual identity?

Setting Goals and Expectations for the Conversation

It's important to set goals and expectations for the conversation with your child. This can help you stay focused and ensure that you cover all the topics you want to address. Some goals to consider include:

- Providing accurate and age-appropriate information

- Creating a safe and supportive environment for the conversation

- Encouraging open and honest communication

- Promoting healthy attitudes towards sex and relationships

Remember, preparing yourself for the conversation is just as important as preparing your child. By dealing with your own discomfort and anxieties, identifying your values and beliefs about sex, and setting goals and expectations, you can create a positive and meaningful conversation with your child.

Once you've prepared yourself for the conversation, it's time to initiate it with your child. In this chapter, we'll explore how to choose the right time and place, start with an open-ended question, and practice active listening and responding to your child's questions and concerns.


It's important to choose the right time and place for the conversation. Here are some things to consider:

- Privacy: Choose a place where you and your child can have privacy and won't be interrupted.

- Time: Choose a time when both you and your child are relaxed and not distracted by other activities.

- Age-appropriateness: Consider your child's age and developmental level when choosing the time and place. For example, younger children may be more comfortable talking while doing an activity, like playing with toys or going for a walk.



Starting the conversation with an open-ended question can help encourage your child to share their thoughts and feelings. Here are some examples of open-ended questions to start the conversation:

- "What do you know about sex?"

- "Have you heard any words or phrases that you don't understand?"

- "Do you have any questions about how babies are made?"

Remember to be patient and allow your child time to respond. Don't be afraid to ask follow-up questions or provide clarification if needed.



Active listening is an important part of any conversation, and it's especially important when talking to your child about sex. Here are some tips for active listening:

- Focus on your child: Give your child your full attention and avoid distractions.

- Validate their feelings: Let your child know that it's okay to feel uncomfortable or embarrassed about the topic.

- Respond with honesty and accuracy: Provide accurate and age-appropriate information in response to your child's questions.

Remember to remain calm and supportive, even if your child asks a difficult or unexpected question. Use the conversation as an opportunity to reinforce your child's self-esteem and promote healthy attitudes towards sex and relationships.

In conclusion, initiating the conversation with your child about sex can be a daunting task, but it's an important step in promoting their sexual health and well-being. By choosing the right time and place, starting with an open-ended question, and practicing active listening and responding to your child's questions and concerns, you can create a safe and supportive environment for this important conversation.

Now that you've initiated the conversation with your child about sex, it's time to delve into specific topics. In this chapter, we'll explore how to address specific topics such as puberty and physical changes, sexual anatomy and function, gender and sexual orientation, relationships and dating, consent and boundaries, and safe sex and contraception.

## Puberty and Physical Changes

Puberty is a natural and normal part of development, but it can be a challenging time for both parents and children. Here are some tips for discussing puberty and physical changes with your child:

- Use appropriate language: Use age-appropriate and anatomically correct language when discussing puberty and physical changes.

- Normalize physical changes: Let your child know that physical changes are a normal part of development.

- Emphasize self-care: Encourage your child to take care of their body during puberty, such as practicing good hygiene and getting enough rest.

## Sexual Anatomy and Function

Discussing sexual anatomy and function can be uncomfortable, but it's important for your child to have a basic understanding of their body. Here are some tips for addressing sexual anatomy and function:

- Use age-appropriate language: Use age-appropriate language when discussing sexual anatomy and function.

- Emphasize safety and health: Discuss the importance of hygiene, safety, and health when it comes to sexual activity.

- Provide accurate information: Provide accurate information about sexual anatomy and function, while keeping in mind your child's age and developmental level.

## Gender and Sexual Orientation

As children grow and develop, they may have questions about gender and sexual orientation. Here are some tips for discussing gender and sexual orientation with your child:

- Use inclusive language: Use language that is inclusive of all gender identities and sexual orientations.

- Encourage acceptance: Encourage your child to accept and respect people of all gender identities and sexual orientations.

- Emphasize individuality: Let your child know that it's okay to be themselves, regardless of their gender identity or sexual orientation.

## Relationships and Dating

As your child gets older, they may begin to explore relationships and dating. Here are some tips for discussing relationships and dating with your child:

- Emphasize respect: Discuss the importance of respect, communication, and consent in relationships.

- Encourage healthy relationships: Encourage your child to seek out healthy relationships that are built on mutual trust and respect.

- Discuss boundaries: Discuss the importance of setting and respecting personal boundaries in relationships.

## Consent and Boundaries

Consent and boundaries are important topics to discuss with your child, especially as they enter adolescence. Here are some tips for discussing consent and boundaries with your child:

- Define consent: Define consent and discuss the importance of asking for and giving consent in all types of relationships.

- Discuss personal boundaries: Discuss the importance of setting and respecting personal boundaries in all types of relationships.

- Emphasize communication: Encourage your child to communicate their boundaries and respect the boundaries of others.

As your child grows and begins to explore sexual activity, it's important to discuss safe sex and contraception. Here are some tips for discussing safe sex and contraception with your child:

- Emphasize safety: Discuss the importance of using condoms and other forms of contraception to prevent sexually transmitted infections and unintended pregnancy.

- Discuss options: Discuss the different types of contraception available and encourage your child to talk to their healthcare provider about what option is best for them.

- Encourage open communication: Encourage your child to talk to their partner about their sexual history and use of contraception.

In conclusion, addressing specific topics related to sex education can be challenging, but it's an important step in promoting your child's sexual health and well-being.

As you talk to your child about sex, you may encounter challenging situations that require special attention. In this chapter, we'll explore how to navigate situations such as dealing with resistance or discomfort from your child, handling questions you may not know the answer to, and addressing conflicting messages from media and peers.

## Dealing with Resistance or Discomfort from Your Child

It's common for children to feel uncomfortable or resistant when talking about sex. Here are some tips for navigating these situations:

- Normalize discomfort: Let your child know that it's normal to feel uncomfortable or resistant when talking about sex, but that it's an important conversation to have.

How to Talk to Your Child About Sex

- Take a break: If your child becomes overwhelmed or resistant during the conversation, take a break and come back to it later when they're ready.

- Validate their feelings: Validate your child's feelings and let them know that it's okay to have questions and concerns.

## Handling Questions You May Not Know the Answer To

It's natural to feel unsure or unprepared when your child asks a question you don't know the answer to. Here are some tips for handling these situations:

- Admit when you don't know: If you're unsure of the answer to a question, admit it and offer to research the topic together.

- Use resources: Utilize reputable resources such as books, websites, or healthcare providers to help answer your child's questions.

- Encourage critical thinking: Encourage your child to think critically about the information they receive and to ask questions when they're unsure.

## Addressing Conflicting Messages from Media and Peers

Children may receive conflicting messages about sex from media and peers, which can be confusing. Here are some tips for addressing these conflicting messages:

- Discuss media messages: Discuss the messages your child sees in the media and how they may not always be accurate or healthy.

- Encourage healthy relationships: Encourage your child to seek out healthy relationships that are built on respect and communication.

- Provide accurate information: Provide your child with accurate information about sex and relationships, while emphasizing the importance of critical thinking and questioning.

In conclusion, navigating challenging situations when talking to your child about sex is an important part of promoting their sexual health and well-being. By normalizing discomfort, admitting when you don't know the answer, and encouraging critical thinking, you can help your child navigate these situations with confidence and ease.

Creating a Healthy and Positive Attitude towards Sex

Talking to your child about sex is not only about providing them with accurate information; it's also about promoting healthy attitudes towards sex. In this chapter, we'll explore how to encourage self-respect and respect for others, foster open communication, and promote a healthy and positive attitude towards sex.

# PROMOTING HEALTHY ATTITUDES TOWARDS SEX

Promoting healthy attitudes towards sex starts with modeling positive behaviors and attitudes. Here are some ways to promote healthy attitudes towards sex:

- Emphasize the importance of consent: Discuss the importance of obtaining explicit consent and respecting boundaries in all sexual situations.

- Promote healthy relationships: Encourage your child to seek out healthy relationships that are built on respect, communication, and shared values.

- Emphasize the importance of pleasure: Discuss the importance of pleasure and enjoyment in sexual experiences, and how it should be a mutual experience.

Encouraging Self-Respect and Respect for Others

## Encouraging Self-Respect and Respect for Others

Teaching your child to respect themselves and others is a crucial part of promoting healthy attitudes towards sex. Here are some ways to encourage self-respect and respect for others:

- Emphasize the importance of self-respect: Discuss the importance of valuing oneself and setting boundaries that protect their emotional and physical well-being.

- Discuss the importance of respecting others: Discuss how to respect others' boundaries, choices, and decisions, and how to communicate effectively in sexual situations.

## Fostering Open Communication and Ongoing Dialogue

Fostering open communication and ongoing dialogue is key to promoting a healthy and positive attitude towards sex. Here are some ways to foster open communication and ongoing dialogue:

- Create a safe and non-judgmental environment: Create a safe and non-judgmental environment where your child can ask questions, share their thoughts and feelings, and express their concerns without fear of judgment.

- Encourage ongoing dialogue: Encourage ongoing dialogue by checking in with your child regularly, initiating conversations about sex and relationships, and being open to their questions and concerns.

- Normalize open communication: Normalize open communication by emphasizing that it's healthy and normal to talk about sex and relationships, and that it's important to do so in a respectful and open manner.

In conclusion, promoting healthy attitudes towards sex is essential for promoting your child's sexual health and well-being. By emphasizing the importance of consent, promoting healthy relationships, encouraging self-respect and respect for others, and fostering open communication and ongoing dialogue, you can help your child develop a healthy and positive attitude towards sex.

CONCLUSION

In this book, we have discussed the importance of talking to your child about sex, addressing common fears and misconceptions, and providing strategies for initiating conversations about sex. We have also explored the basics of sex education, how to approach difficult topics such as consent and safe sex, and how to navigate challenging situations.

As parents, it's important to understand that talking to your child about sex is not a one-time event. Rather, it's an ongoing conversation that should be revisited as your child grows and develops. By having ongoing conversations about sex, you can help your child develop a healthy and positive attitude towards sex, make informed decisions, and ultimately promote their sexual health and well-being.

Recap of Key Points and Strategies

How to Talk to Your Child About Sex

Throughout this book, we have covered many key points and strategies for talking to your child about sex. Here are some of the most important:

- Start early and have ongoing conversations about sex.

- Approach the conversation with openness and honesty.

- Listen actively and respond to your child's questions and concerns.

- Address specific topics such as puberty, sexual anatomy and function, gender and sexual orientation, relationships and dating, consent and boundaries, and safe sex and contraception.

- Foster open communication and ongoing dialogue by creating a safe and non-judgmental environment.

- Promote healthy attitudes towards sex by emphasizing the importance of consent, healthy relationships, pleasure, self-respect, and respect for others.

Encouragement and Support for Parents

As a parent, talking to your child about sex can be challenging and uncomfortable. However, it's important to remember that you are not alone in this journey. Many resources are available to support you, including books, online resources, and professional counseling.

Remember, the most important thing is to be there for your child, listen to their questions and concerns, and provide accurate information in a safe and non-judgmental environment. By doing so, you can help your child develop a healthy and positive attitude towards sex and ultimately promote their sexual health and well-being.